Cognitive Rehabilitation Therapy for Traumatic Brain Injury

Model Study Protocols and Frameworks to Advance the State of the Science

Workshop Summary

Karin Matchett, *Rapporteur*

Board on the Health of Select Populations

INSTITUTE OF MEDICINE
OF THE NATIONAL ACADEMIES

THE NATIONAL ACADEMIES PRESS
Washington, D.C.
www.nap.edu

THE NATIONAL ACADEMIES PRESS   500 Fifth Street, NW   Washington, DC 20001

NOTICE: The workshop that is the subject of this workshop summary was approved by the Governing Board of the National Research Council, whose members are drawn from the councils of the National Academy of Sciences, the National Academy of Engineering, and the Institute of Medicine.

This activity was supported by Contract No. HHSP23320042509XI/HHSP23337029T/0002 between the National Academy of Sciences and the U.S. Department of Health and Human Services. The views presented in this publication do not necessarily reflect the views of the organizations or agencies that provided support for the activity.

International Standard Book Number-13:   978-0-309-26786-1
International Standard Book Number-10:   0-309-26786-2

Additional copies of this report are available for sale from the National Academies Press, 500 Fifth Street, NW, Keck 360, Washington, DC 20001; (800) 624-6242 or (202) 334-3313; http://www.nap.edu.

For more information about the Institute of Medicine, visit the IOM home page at: www.iom.edu.

Copyright 2013 by the National Academy of Sciences. All rights reserved.

Printed in the United States of America

The serpent has been a symbol of long life, healing, and knowledge among almost all cultures and religions since the beginning of recorded history. The serpent adopted as a logotype by the Institute of Medicine is a relief carving from ancient Greece, now held by the Staatliche Museen in Berlin.

Suggested citation: IOM (Institute of Medicine). 2013. *Cognitive rehabilitation therapy for traumatic brain injury: Model study protocols and frameworks to advance the state of the science: Workshop summary.* Washington, DC: The National Academies Press.

*"Knowing is not enough; we must apply.
Willing is not enough; we must do."*
—Goethe

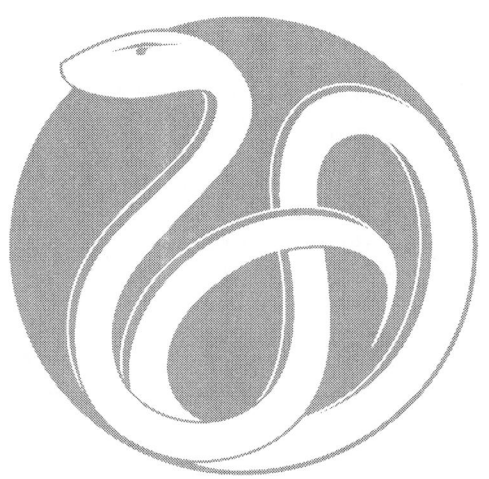

INSTITUTE OF MEDICINE
OF THE NATIONAL ACADEMIES

Advising the Nation. Improving Health.

THE NATIONAL ACADEMIES
Advisers to the Nation on Science, Engineering, and Medicine

The **National Academy of Sciences** is a private, nonprofit, self-perpetuating society of distinguished scholars engaged in scientific and engineering research, dedicated to the furtherance of science and technology and to their use for the general welfare. Upon the authority of the charter granted to it by the Congress in 1863, the Academy has a mandate that requires it to advise the federal government on scientific and technical matters. Dr. Ralph J. Cicerone is president of the National Academy of Sciences.

The **National Academy of Engineering** was established in 1964, under the charter of the National Academy of Sciences, as a parallel organization of outstanding engineers. It is autonomous in its administration and in the selection of its members, sharing with the National Academy of Sciences the responsibility for advising the federal government. The National Academy of Engineering also sponsors engineering programs aimed at meeting national needs, encourages education and research, and recognizes the superior achievements of engineers. Dr. Charles M. Vest is president of the National Academy of Engineering.

The **Institute of Medicine** was established in 1970 by the National Academy of Sciences to secure the services of eminent members of appropriate professions in the examination of policy matters pertaining to the health of the public. The Institute acts under the responsibility given to the National Academy of Sciences by its congressional charter to be an adviser to the federal government and, upon its own initiative, to identify issues of medical care, research, and education. Dr. Harvey V. Fineberg is president of the Institute of Medicine.

The **National Research Council** was organized by the National Academy of Sciences in 1916 to associate the broad community of science and technology with the Academy's purposes of furthering knowledge and advising the federal government. Functioning in accordance with general policies determined by the Academy, the Council has become the principal operating agency of both the National Academy of Sciences and the National Academy of Engineering in providing services to the government, the public, and the scientific and engineering communities. The Council is administered jointly by both Academies and the Institute of Medicine. Dr. Ralph J. Cicerone and Dr. Charles M. Vest are chair and vice chair, respectively, of the National Research Council.

www.national-academies.org

PLANNING COMMITTEE ON COGNITIVE REHABILITATION
THERAPY FOR TRAUMATIC BRAIN INJURY:
MODEL STUDY PROTOCOLS AND FRAMEWORKS
TO ADVANCE THE STATE OF THE SCIENCE[1]

IRA SHOULSON (*Chair*), Professor of Neurology, Pharmacology and Human Science, and Director of the Program for Regulatory Science and Medicine, Georgetown University, Washington, DC
RICHARD KEEFE, Professor of Psychiatry and Behavioral Sciences, Duke University Medical Center, Durham, NC
MARY R. T. KENNEDY, Associate Professor, Department of Speech-Language-Hearing Science, University of Minnesota, Minneapolis
HILAIRE THOMPSON, Assistant Professor in the School of Nursing, University of Washington, Seattle
JOHN WHYTE, Director, Moss Rehabilitation Research Institute, Elkins Park, PA

Consultant

BARBARA G. VICKREY, Professor and Vice Chair, Department of Neurology, University of California, Los Angeles

IOM Staff

REBECCA KOEHLER, Program Officer
MARYJO M. OSTER, Program Officer
JON Q. SANDERS, Program Associate
ANDREA COHEN, Financial Associate
FREDERICK (RICK) ERDTMANN, Director, Board on the Health of Select Populations

---

[1] Institute of Medicine planning committees are solely responsible for organizing the workshop, identifying topics, and choosing speakers. The responsibility for the published workshop summary rests with the workshop rapporteur and the institution.

Reviewers

This workshop summary has been reviewed in draft form by individuals chosen for their diverse perspectives and technical expertise, in accordance with procedures approved by the National Research Council's Report Review Committee. The purpose of this independent review is to provide candid and critical comments that will assist the institution in making its published workshop summary as sound as possible and to ensure that the workshop summary meets institutional standards for objectivity, evidence, and responsiveness to the study charge. The review comments and draft manuscript remain confidential to protect the integrity of the process. We wish to thank the following individuals for their review of this workshop summary:

Alison Cernich, Defense Centers of Excellence
Wayne A. Gordon, Mount Sinai School of Medicine
Mary V. Radomski, Sister Kenny Research Center
Rodney Vanderploeg, James A. Haley VA Hospital

Although the reviewers listed above have provided many constructive comments and suggestions, they did not see the final draft of the workshop summary before its release. The review of this workshop summary was overseen by **Jack C. Ebeler,** Health Policy Alternatives, Inc. Appointed by the Institute of Medicine, he was responsible for making certain that an independent examination of this workshop summary was carried out in accordance with institutional procedures and that all review comments were carefully considered. Responsibility for the final content of this workshop summary rests entirely with the rapporteur and the institution.

Acknowledgments

Many individuals were responsible for the planning of the workshop and the production of this summary. We wish to additionally thank Charles Drebing for his assistance and expertise.

Contents

1 INTRODUCTION 1
Objectives of the Workshop, 2
Organization of This Summary, 3

2 OVERVIEW OF THE INSTITUTE OF MEDICINE REPORT
(OCTOBER 2011) 5
The Committee's Approach, 6
Analysis of the 90 Studies, 8
Example of the Committee's Process, 9
Overall Findings from the Analysis of the Literature, 10
The Limitations of the Current Literature on CRT for TBI, 10
The Committee's Conclusions, 11

3 THE TRANSLATIONAL PIPELINE AND CLASSIFICATION
SCHEMES FOR CRT INTERVENTIONS 13
The Translational Pipeline, 13
Guidelines for Creating Meaningful Descriptions of CRT
Interventions, 22

4 KEY THEMES 27
The Translational Pipeline and Research Design, 28
Severity Levels of TBI: Discussion of Mild Injury, 30
Components of Research Studies and Their Characteristics at
Different Points in the Maturational Process, 32

Databases, 38
Who Owns This Process Going Forward?, 39
Closing Remarks, 42

REFERENCES 45

APPENDIXES

A Recommendations of the IOM Report *Cognitive Rehabilitation Therapy for Traumatic Brain Injury: Evaluating the Evidence* 47
B Workshop Agenda 51
C Biosketches of the Workshop Speakers and Moderators 55

1

Introduction

In October 2011, the Institute of Medicine (IOM) released the report *Cognitive Rehabilitation Therapy for Traumatic Brain Injury: Evaluating the Evidence*, assessing the published evidence for the effectiveness of using cognitive rehabilitation therapy (CRT) to treat people with traumatic brain injury (TBI) (see Box 1-1 for a statement of task for the report). TBI has gained increasing attention in the past 15 years because of its status as the signature wound of American military conflicts in Iraq and Afghanistan (DVBIC, 2011; Snell and Halter, 2010). Growing numbers of U.S. service members are suffering traumatic brain injuries and are surviving them, given that (a) the majority of traumatic brain injuries are mild and (b) life-saving measures for more severe injuries have significantly improved. People with any level of injury can require ongoing health care in their recovery, helping them to regain (or compensate for) their losses of function and supporting their full integration into their social structure and an improved quality of life.

One form of treatment for TBI is CRT, a systematic, goal-oriented approach to helping patients overcome cognitive impairments. The Department of Defense (DoD) asked the IOM to evaluate CRT for traumatic brain injury in order to guide the DoD's use and coverage in the Military Health System. *Cognitive Rehabilitation Therapy for Traumatic Brain Injury: Evaluating the Evidence* was the IOM's resulting study of the evidence. The report's conclusions revolved around the fact that there is little continuity among research studies of the effectiveness of different types of CRT, and there exist only small amounts of evidence (or, in many cases, none) demonstrating the effectiveness of using CRT to treat TBI—although

> **BOX 1-1**
> **Statement of Task for the Committee That Authored** *Cognitive Rehabilitation Therapy for Traumatic Brain Injury: Evaluating the Evidence*
>
> A consensus committee shall design and perform a methodology to review, synthesize, and assess the salient literature and determine if there exists sufficient evidence for effective treatment using cognitive rehabilitation therapy (CRT) for three categories of traumatic brain injury (TBI) severity—mild, moderate, and severe—and will also consider the evidence across three phases of recovery—acute, subacute, and chronic. In assessing CRT treatment efficacy, the committee will consider comparison groups such as no treatment, sham treatment, or other non-pharmacological treatment. The committee will determine the effects of specific CRT treatment on improving (1) attention, (2) language and communication, (3) memory, (4) visuospatial perception, and (5) executive function (e.g., problem solving and awareness). The committee will also evaluate the use of multi-modal CRT in improving cognitive function as well as the available scientific evidence on the safety and efficacy of CRT when applied using telehealth technology devices. The committee will further evaluate evidence relating CRT's effectiveness on the family and family training. The goal of this evaluation is to identify specific CRT interventions with sufficient evidence base to support their widespread use in the MHS, including coverage through the TRICARE benefit.
>
> The committee shall gather and analyze data and information that addresses:
>
> 1. a comprehensive literature review of studies conducted, including but not limited to studies conducted on MHS or VA wounded warriors;
> 2. an assessment of current evidence supporting the effectiveness of specific CRT interventions in specific deficits associated with moderate and severe TBI;
> 3. an assessment of current evidence supporting the effectiveness of specific CRT interventions in specific deficits associated with mild TBI;
> 4. an assessment of (1) the state of practice of CRT and (2) whether requirements for training, education and experience for providers outside the MHS direct-care system to deliver the identified evidence-based interventions are sufficient to ensure reasonable, consistent quality of care across the United States; and
> 5. an independent assessment of the treatment of traumatic brain injury by cognitive rehabilitation therapy within the MHS if time or resources permit.

the evidence that *does* exist generally indicates that CRT interventions have some effectiveness.

OBJECTIVES OF THE WORKSHOP

The workshop brought together experts in health services administration, research, and clinical practice from the civilian and military arenas in order to discuss the barriers for evaluating the effectiveness of CRT care and for identifying suggested taxonomy, terminology, timing, and ways forward for CRT researchers. The workshop consisted of individuals and was not intended to constitute a comprehensive group. Select decision makers in the Military Health System and Veterans Affairs (VA) and researchers were invited to participate. The workshop was designed to spur thinking about (1) the types of research necessary to move the field forward toward evidence-based clinical guidelines, (2) what the translational pipeline looks like and what its current deficiencies are, and (3) considerations that decision makers may choose to use as they decide what research they will support and decide how they will balance the urgency of the need with the level of evidence for CRT interventions.

Warren Lockette, Chief Medical Officer for TRICARE, offered a perspective from the DoD aimed to guide the workshop discussions toward DoD's primary challenges in its efforts to help service members suffering from TBIs. He described how the Military Health System's coverage of CRT treatments is in need of a portfolio of interventions whose effectiveness has been scientifically determined. Slightly upstream is the pressing need of DoD program managers, who would greatly benefit from a clear understanding of the major research needs that must be met in order for the DoD to obtain such a portfolio of proven interventions. The DoD seeks scientifically based guidance about what CRT interventions are effective, and for whom. Lockette emphasized the critical need for research that, while scientifically rigorous, also takes into account the budgetary environment in which CRT treatments are delivered—an environment very cost-constrained. He asked workshop participants to consider what kinds of techniques need to be pursued as part of a research agenda and what the standards for research programs should be to effectively and efficiently move the field toward specific, scientifically based guidance for CRT practitioners charged with helping injured service members regain functionality and improve their quality of life.

ORGANIZATION OF THIS SUMMARY

The workshop consisted of three types of discussion: formal presentations, question/answer periods, and small-group discussions followed by the groups' reporting back and subsequent large-group discussion. Small-group discussions were focused on sets of questions designed by members of the planning committee, and each small-group discussion was moderated by a planning committee member. This document was prepared by rapporteur Karin Matchett for the Board on the Health of Select Populations of the IOM as a factual summary of what occurred at the workshop Cognitive

Rehabilitation Therapy for Traumatic Brain Injury: Model Study Protocols and Frameworks to Advance the State of the Science.

This workshop summary begins with summaries of the three formal presentations: an overview of the original IOM report, *Cognitive Rehabilitation Therapy for Traumatic Brain Injury: Evaluating the Evidence* (Chapter 2), an overview of the translational pipeline for using CRT for TBI, and a discussion about finding optimal ways of describing CRT intervention (both in Chapter 3). Chapter 4 summarizes the suggestions and recommendations of the workshop participants, organized by theme. The recommendations expressed in Chapter 4 are in no way a consensus; rather, they are meant to inform and guide, where relevant or helpful, health services administrators as they map out future research directions and clinical guidelines for using CRT to treat TBI.

In accordance with the policies of the IOM, the summary does not attempt to establish any conclusions or recommendations about needs and future directions, focusing instead on issues identified by the speakers and workshop participants. Whenever possible, ideas presented at the workshop are attributed to the individual who expressed them. Any opinions, conclusions, or recommendations discussed in this workshop summary are solely those of the individual participants and should not be construed as reflecting consensus or endorsement by the workshop, the Board on the Health of Select Populations, the IOM, or the National Academies.

2

Overview of the Institute of Medicine Report (October 2011)

Barbara Vickrey, Professor and Vice Chair of the Department of Neurology, University of California, Los Angeles, began by reiterating two questions that were central to the goals of the workshop: How can the evidence base be strengthened, and how can this process take place in a way that is targeted to what will be most helpful to the health services decision makers? Vickrey went on to summarize the charge to the committee, and its process, findings, and recommendations.

The study took place over 12 months, included two public meetings and four closed meetings, and centered on an extensive literature review. The committee's report, released in October 2011, is divided into two sections: background and assessment of the evidence. The background section investigated definitions and types of traumatic brain injury (TBI), the factors that affect recovery, the definition of cognitive rehabilitation therapy (CRT), an evaluation of the range of interventions that fall under this umbrella, and the state of the practice of CRT.

Vickrey described the committee's efforts to survey the various definitions of CRT as used by professional societies and health care organizations, citing one definition used by the Brain Injury Interdisciplinary Special Interest Group (BI-ISIG):

> Cognitive rehabilitation is a systematic, functionally oriented service of therapeutic cognitive activities, based on an assessment and understanding of the person's brain-behavior deficits. Services are directed to achieve functional changes by (1) reinforcing, strengthening, or reestablishing previously learned patterns of behavior; or (2) establishing new patterns of

cognitive activity or compensatory mechanisms for impaired neurological systems. (Harley et al., 1992)

The committee focused its work around the following question: Do cognitive rehabilitation interventions improve function and reduce cognitive deficits in adults with mild or moderate-severe TBI? The committee was charged with investigating the literature on interventions addressing each major cognitive domain—attention, executive function, language and social communication, visuospatial perception, and memory—as well as multi-modal interventions (CRT that comprehensively targets more than one domain). Within each cognitive domain, the committee looked for research on two severities of injury (mild TBI and moderate-severe TBI) and three stages of recovery (acute, subacute, and chronic). Regarding outcomes, the committee assessed the evidence for immediate benefit and long-term benefit, and investigated whether patient-centered outcomes were assessed—whether studies examined the effects of an intervention on a patient's reintegration into the community or demonstrated improvement in patients' quality of life. The committee also looked for any evidence to suggest that CRT interventions are associated with risk or harm, and the committee examined the safety and efficacy of interventions delivered through "telehealth" technology.

Vickrey presented a model (Figure 2-1) showing the relationship between CRT and the domains affected in a given patient on the one hand, and the desired type of change, outcome in terms of activities, and outcome in terms of broader participation in society on the other.

She highlighted the distinction between restorative and compensatory types of changes, noting that the committee treated these separately in its analysis of the literature. She also highlighted the vast heterogeneity among patients that comes into play during and after an intervention, which strongly influences the delivery of the intervention as well as the outcomes. In particular, comorbidities are very diverse among people suffering from TBI (for example, patients may also have posttraumatic stress disorder, have suffered other nonbrain injuries, or struggle with substance abuse), as are the environments in which patients live. These variables have a strong impact on the effects and success of a CRT intervention.

THE COMMITTEE'S APPROACH

The committee developed a search strategy and applied it to a large number of databases, initially looking at the prior 20 years and then going back selectively to some earlier dates. The initial search yielded 856 published articles. The committee then narrowed the results according to a set of inclusion and exclusion criteria, and included randomized trials

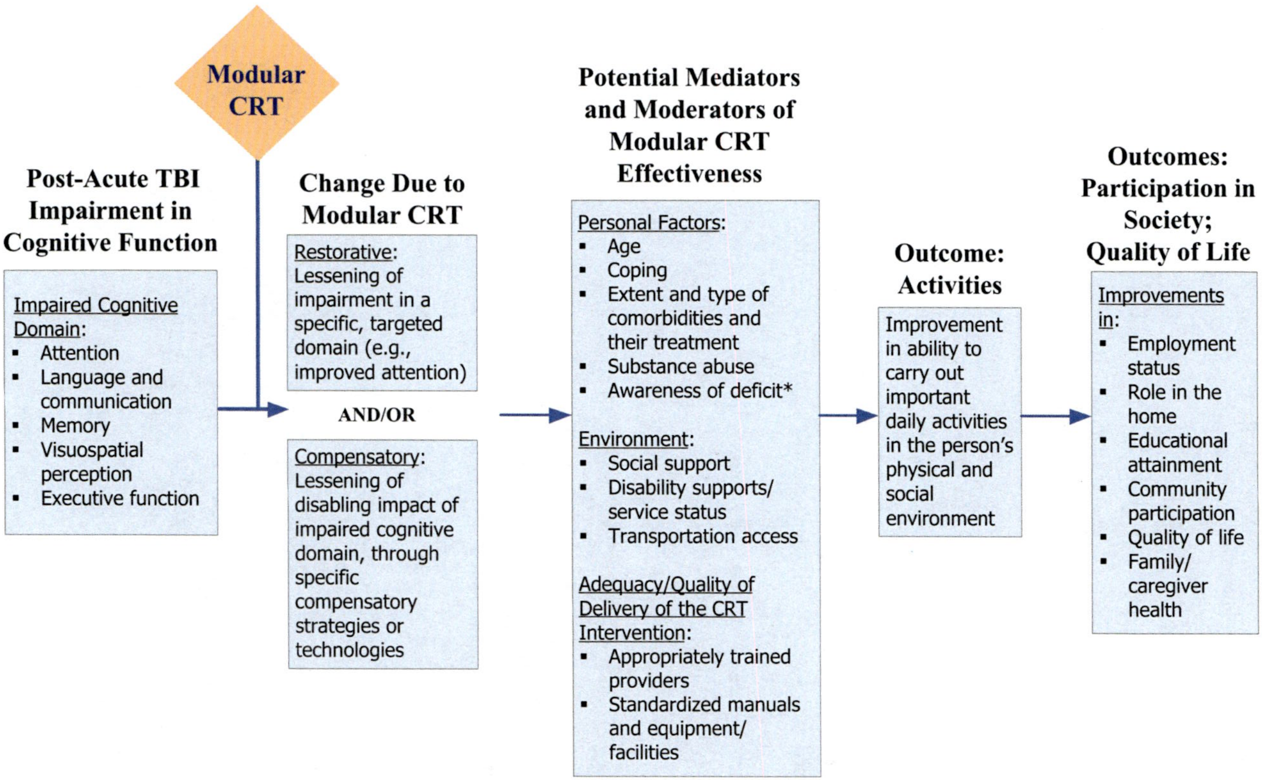

Post-Acute TBI Impairment in Cognitive Function

Impaired Cognitive Domain:
- Attention
- Language and communication
- Memory
- Visuospatial perception
- Executive function

Modular CRT

Change Due to Modular CRT

Restorative: Lessening of impairment in a specific, targeted domain (e.g., improved attention)

AND/OR

Compensatory: Lessening of disabling impact of impaired cognitive domain, through specific compensatory strategies or technologies

Potential Mediators and Moderators of Modular CRT Effectiveness

Personal Factors:
- Age
- Coping
- Extent and type of comorbidities and their treatment
- Substance abuse
- Awareness of deficit*

Environment:
- Social support
- Disability supports/service status
- Transportation access

Adequacy/Quality of Delivery of the CRT Intervention:
- Appropriately trained providers
- Standardized manuals and equipment/facilities

Outcome: Activities

Improvement in ability to carry out important daily activities in the person's physical and social environment

Outcomes: Participation in Society; Quality of Life

Improvements in:
- Employment status
- Role in the home
- Educational attainment
- Community participation
- Quality of life
- Family/caregiver health

FIGURE 2-1 Model for modular CRT intervening between postacute TBI cognitive impairment in a domain, and outcomes.
* For some domains, the CRT intervention may also target deficit awareness, for example, videotape of a social interaction followed by a critique will increase awareness of deficit in language and communication.

(weighted the most heavily), some pre/post studies, nonrandomized comparison groups, and experimental designs based on single subjects with controls, for certain domains. The number of studies in the narrowed group was 90.

ANALYSIS OF THE 90 STUDIES

Each study was reviewed by at least two committee members, who abstracted the key data and applied the committee's agreed-upon grading system to judge the strength of the evidence for a particular intervention for a particular domain and for patients in a particular stage of recovery from a particular severity of brain injury. Evidence was graded according to four categories: none, limited, modest, and strong (Box 2-1). No evidence (0) meant either that no studies were found or that studies existed but were seriously flawed or otherwise very limited. Limited evidence (+) meant that the committee identified either some kind of result from one study or mixed results from two or more studies. Modest evidence (++) signified at least two studies reporting interpretable, informative, and concordant types of results. Strong evidence (+++) signified studies with high-quality study design—reproducible, consistent, large, and having good statistical power.

BOX 2-1
System for Grading the Strength of the Evidence

None or not informative (0)
  No evidence because the intervention has not been studied or uninformative evidence because of null results from flawed or otherwise limited studies
Limited (+)
  Interpretable result from a single study or mixed results from two or more studies
Modest (++)
  Two or more studies reporting interpretable, informative, and largely similar result(s)
Strong (+++)
  Reproducible, consistent, and decisive findings from two or more independent studies characterized by the following:
  - Replication, reflected by the number of studies in the same direction (at least two studies)
  - Statistical power and scope of studies (*N* size of the study and whether it is single-site or multisite)
  - Quality of the study design, meaning its ability to measure appropriate endpoints (to evaluate efficacy and safety) and minimize bias and confounding

The committee prepared narrative and tabular summaries of the evidence on which its deliberations were then based.

EXAMPLE OF THE COMMITTEE'S PROCESS

Vickrey gave a snapshot of the committee's process of assessing the evidence for CRT interventions in one domain, language and social communication. The committee found a total of five studies, of which four were randomized trials (thus given relatively greater weight) and one was a nonrandomized parallel group study. Regarding severity of injury, they found only studies of moderate-severe TBI; no information was found on interventions treating mild injuries. Regarding stage of recovery, the committee found studies only pertaining to the chronic phase. The committee graded the evidence for each study regarding immediate or long-term outcomes and regarding patient-centered outcomes, that is, improved social communication, integration into the community or social functioning in the community, or quality of life more globally.

The committee found a range of levels of evidence of the effectiveness and efficacy of CRT interventions for the various domains. For the domain of language and social communication, they found the evidence for efficacy of CRT interventions regarding patient-centered outcomes to be not informative—no studies investigated this. The committee found the evidence for short-term benefits to be modest for chronic, moderate-severe TBI, based on four randomized clinical trials and one nonrandomized trial. The evidence for long-term benefits was found to be limited for people with chronic, moderate-severe TBI (two randomized clinical trials). Concerning the area where the evidence was modest—that of short-term benefits for chronic, moderate-severe TBI—the efficacious interventions tended to be across small-group outpatient programs employing a standardized protocol for social communication skills training. Appropriate candidates were people who had demonstrated deficits and sufficient capacity to participate in a group program.

Vickrey highlighted an important gap in the process of bringing research results to bear on clinical practice—the lack of dissemination of the studies' details and findings. Where are those protocols posted? Where are the manuals? Where are the description and the tools that a practitioner would need if he or she wanted to deliver that intervention? Vickrey noted that some researchers post them while others do not. She described a need for the protocols and manuals to be made publicly available in order to allow others to deliver a given intervention in a larger population, either as a delivered intervention in treatment programs or for further study.

For some domains there was literature on both mild and moderate-severe TBI, while in others the literature focused on moderate-severe TBI.

Likewise, for some domains there existed studies of both subacute and chronic stages of recovery, while for others there were studies only of the chronic phase. Overall, the committee's review showed that often where there was evidence of benefit, it was in the immediate treatment effect. Fewer studies looked at long-term effects or at patient-centered outcomes.

Regarding study design, Vickrey cited a type of study the committee encountered in which two CRT interventions were compared, but neither was standard of care and neither had been assessed independently to determine its efficacy. The committee had to set the studies aside because they lacked the appropriate comparisons that would have allowed conclusions to be drawn about the effectiveness of the interventions.

OVERALL FINDINGS FROM THE ANALYSIS OF THE LITERATURE

Vickrey explained that the literature signals evidence of some benefit of certain forms of CRT for TBI, evidence that varies across cognitive domains. The evidence is insufficient overall to provide definitive guidance for translation into clinical practice guidelines, particularly in selecting the most effective treatment(s) for a particular patient. The committee found very little evidence of adverse effects or harm associated with CRT, but it recommended that future studies assess such risks. And, the overall evidence is insufficient to clearly establish whether telehealth technology delivery modes are more or less effective or more or less safe than other means of delivering CRT.

THE LIMITATIONS OF THE CURRENT LITERATURE ON CRT FOR TBI

Vickrey discussed how the limitations of the extant body of research centered on two areas: the lack of sufficient standardization and comparability, and the lack of sufficiently powered trials. Regarding standardization, there is a need for studies to take into account the heterogeneity of patient demographics, "active ingredients" of CRT interventions, and outcome measures. In particular, she emphasized the importance of precisely describing the hypothesized active ingredients. Regarding statistical power, she noted that many studies were at the pilot stage and were not followed up with more powerful study designs that would advance the knowledge gained about a specific intervention and move it toward clinical usefulness. Even the most promising treatments lacked sufficiently powered trials to answer practical questions about (1) the relationships between patient characteristics and responses to certain treatments, (2) the lasting benefits of treatments that have positive results in the short term, and (3) how or whether treatments affect patients' real-world tasks, community integration, and quality of life. Subsequent studies to delve into these variables do not exist. She noted also a serious need for a plan to follow through on signals detected in early studies.

THE COMMITTEE'S CONCLUSIONS

Vickrey emphasized that the committee's conclusion that the evidence was limited signified only that the *amount* of evidence was limited. The *type* of evidence of the effectiveness of CRT for TBI was often tilted in its favor. There were definitely signals of benefit, but there was not enough information to confidently declare a generalizable benefit for any specific intervention.

The committee supported the ongoing application of CRT for TBI. Crucially, it recommended building on the literature base and considering how to design studies that build on the existing signal and strengthen the evidence to the point that it becomes useful for health services decision makers.

3

The Translational Pipeline and Classification Schemes for CRT Interventions

THE TRANSLATIONAL PIPELINE

John Whyte, Director of Moss Rehabilitation Research Institute, discussed his view of clinical research as a developmental process, how the translational pipeline referred to throughout medicine applies to cognitive rehabilitation therapy (CRT) for traumatic brain injury (TBI), and where and why the translational pipeline often gets bogged down. He characterized the translational pipeline as a maturational process, one in which early studies identify a signal and are built upon by later studies that increasingly solidify the evidence and that make the use of cognitive rehabilitation therapies more practical and ultimately cost-effective. Regarding the committee's scoring methodology, he reiterated that the scores of one plus (+) and two plusses (++) signaled not always a weak effect, but the fact that research on the interventions was at an early point in a maturational process.

The Traditional, Pharmaceutical Model of Translation

Whyte defined translational research as translating the findings of basic research into medical practice and thus meaningful health outcomes, and he began by outlining the pharmaceutical model of translation and its progression through several phases of research, noting the ways that behavioral therapy is similar or different. He described how pharmaceutically based translational research follows a relatively rigid series of steps that have different sample sizes and different typical research designs, and that are designed to answer different research problems as the maturational process proceeds. He began with an implicit Phase 0 of idea generation, based, for example, on results from an animal model or designer drug. Phase I involves research on safety and identifying doses, generally in a small number of subjects. Phase II is proof of principle, usually a single-site clinical trial with or without a control group, depending on the natural history of the condition being studied. Phase III looks at efficacy and commonly takes the form of a multicenter randomized clinical trial. Phase IV investigates effectiveness of the drug using postmarketing surveillance.

This model serves drug development well, for example, by delaying costly research in large numbers of humans until basic safety and efficacy have been established. In contrast, Whyte noted the ways in which research on CRT is less linear and more complex. First, idea generation originates from a wide range of areas, for example, basic neuroscience, different patient populations, and engineering and studies of compensatory strategies and devices. Second, regarding safety and dose finding, dose-related toxicity is less of a factor than for drug trials; instead, the question of doses is one of impact. This means that studies often examine efficacy earlier in the maturational process than is typical with drug studies. Third, researchers must carry out proof of principle: does the intervention have the intended treatment outcome with respect to the object of treatment? Then come studies to test large-scale efficacy. Studies are broadened to test whether—when the intervention is delivered by a large group of practitioners to a larger group of patients—it still has the intended treatment outcome. Lastly, researchers study an intervention's effectiveness. What meaningful benefit accrues to patients, their ability to function well in society, and their quality of life?

Whyte highlighted a number of elements of the definition of translational research as translating the findings of basic research into medical practice and thus meaningful health outcomes. *Basic research* encompasses not just the typical understanding of basic research as dealing with the cellular level, but also basic cognitive science. *Medical practice* involves assessing both cognitive status and interventions used. *Meaningful health outcomes* spans impacts of interest to a wide range of individuals including the patient, his or her caregivers and social support networks, payers of the health care, and policy makers.

Obstacles to Translation

Looking again at the Phases 0 to IV of translational pipeline, Whyte discussed the nodes at which translation can stall (Figure 3-1). He cited little risk of stalling at Phase 0, which includes idea generation and natural history studies of the clinical condition. The first potential obstacle comes at the point of adapting early studies to human use—assessing safety and carrying out proof-of-principle studies. Accomplishing this is often an itera-

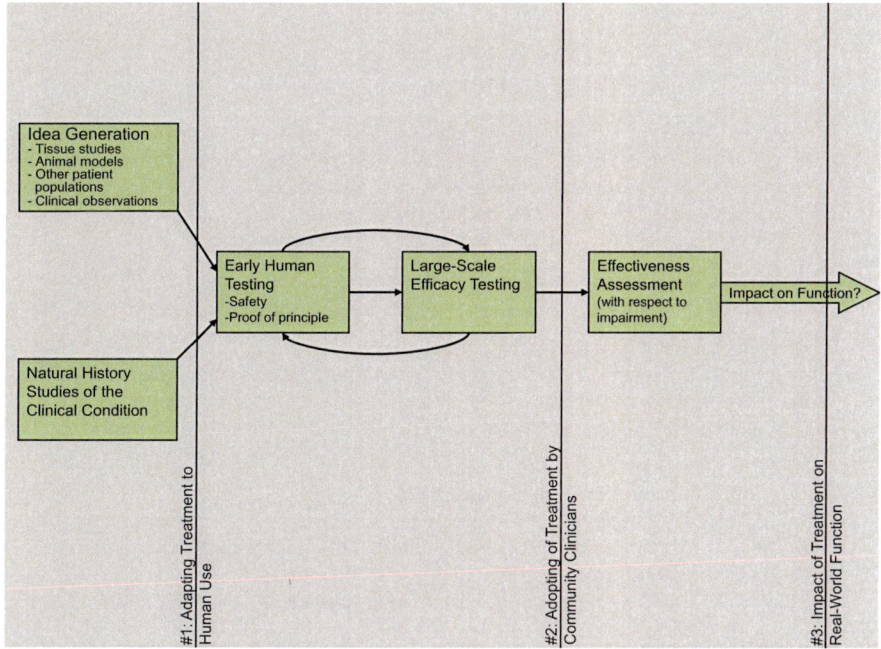

FIGURE 3-1 The translational pipeline and potential barriers to translation.
SOURCE: Whyte presentation.

tive process, looping from early human testing to large-scale efficacy testing and back again, as the research narrows in on an efficacious intervention. Once evidence of efficacy has been established, a second barrier emerges: to assess effectiveness involves creating and assessing behavior change among clinicians, a potentially difficult task. A final obstacle is determining whether the improvement of a specific impairment has practical utility, and if so, to whom?

Treatment Theory and Enablement Theory

Whyte discussed two types of theories related to human function: treatment theory and enablement theory (Box 3-1). Treatment theory specifies the mechanism by which a proposed treatment affects its immediate treatment target, defining the essential ingredients of the treatment that are required to effect the change in the object. The effect of the treatment may be moderated by additional active ingredients, but the essential ingredient

> **BOX 3-1**
> **Theoretical Frameworks for CRT for TBI**
>
> **Treatment Theory**
> A theory that specifies the mechanism by which a proposed treatment changes its immediate treatment target, defining the essential ingredients of the treatment that are required to effect the change in the object.
>
> **Enablement Theory**
> A theory that specifies the causal interrelationships among variables at different levels in the International Classification of Functioning Disability and Health.
>
> **Treatment Object and Treatment Target**
> A treatment object, a component of treatment theory, is the immediate (proximal) outcome of an intervention. A treatment target, a component of enablement theory, is a clinically important treatment outcome and is often distal to the treatment object.
>
> **Active Ingredient and Essential Ingredient**
> An essential ingredient is the component of a treatment that the treatment must have in order to make a predicted change in the treatment object. An active ingredient is a component of a treatment that also moderates the treatment's effect but that is not, itself, required for the treatment to change the treatment object.
>
> **Mechanism of Action**
> The means by which an essential ingredient brings about a change in the treatment object.

is what defines the treatment and distinguishes it from other treatments.[1] In rehabilitation, the set of treatment theories is heterogeneous, with theories hailing from a wide range of fields including physiology, social theory, bioengineering, and many others.

To illustrate the use of a treatment theory and the clarity that it can offer, Whyte gave examples of CRT treatments as well as familiar, physical treatments. He described the use of progressive resistance exercises to increase muscle strength. In this case, the object of the treatment is to increase muscle strength or torque, and in order to accomplish that—the part played by the essential ingredient—there must be repetitive contraction of the muscle and an increasing load. The use of a treatment theory dictates

---
[1] There may exist a difference between Whyte's terminology and terminology more commonly used among CRT researchers. Whyte used "essential" and "active" ingredients according to the above definitions; however, during much of the workshop discussion the participants used "active ingredient" seemingly as the equivalent of Whyte's "essential ingredient."

that the treatment be defined not in terms of the specific intervention, but in terms of the essential ingredient. In this example, the treatment is not defined in terms of the specific manipulations, but rather in terms of the use of any manipulation that involves repetitive contraction of the muscle and an increasing load. All treatments that do those two things would be considered the same treatment. Examples from CRT include neutral cues for goal neglect and hemi-dressing training.

Enablement Theory

Whyte described enablement theory, which addresses the causal relationships among variables at different levels in the International Classification of Functioning Disability and Health (ICF), which separates function into several levels, including tissue, organ function, and personal activity, and social integration (Figure 3-2). Each functional level has a different level of analysis and different attributes, and each is covered by treatment and/or enablement theory.

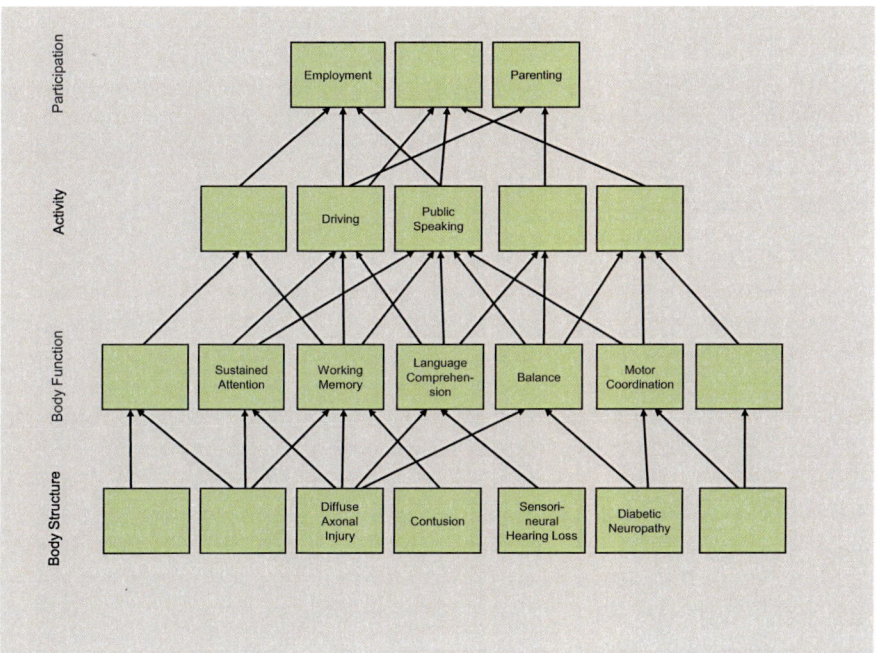

FIGURE 3-2 Enablement theory.
SOURCE: Whyte presentation.

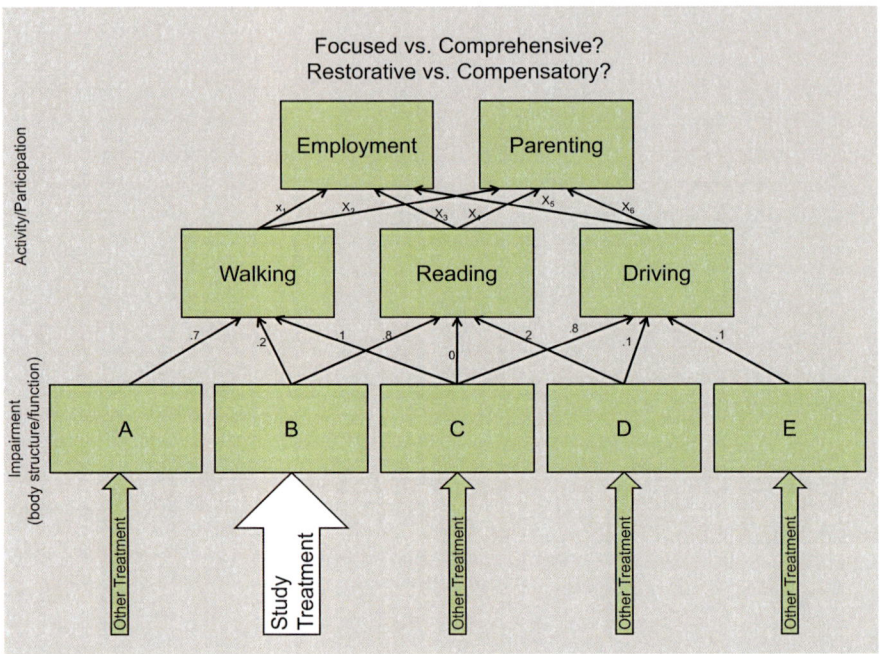

FIGURE 3-3 The intervention under study in the context of the enablement theory. Example of relationship among variables in International Classification of Functioning Disability and Health framework, at impairment (body structure/function) and activity/participation levels.
SOURCE: Whyte presentation.

Enablement theories pose a bigger-picture question: If we improve a particular impairment, what effects will that have elsewhere in this system of human functioning? The outcome of an enablement theory is a *treatment target*, a clinically important treatment outcome that is often distal from (removed or more complex than) the more immediate treatment object.

Enablement theory specifies the location of the arrows (see Figure 3-3) between different levels of pathology and impaired function, as well as the arrows' relative weight. Enablement theory produces conceptual models that take into account the complex interrelationships between more basic types of functioning, such as sustained attention or good motor coordination, and higher-level functioning, such as holding down a job or parenting a child. With enablement theory, a higher-level function can be broken down into lower-level functional components.

Whyte described how treatment theory and enablement theory can bring distinct and complementary tools to a research agenda.

Treatment theory constrains the definition of a treatment, informs researchers' understanding of what kinds of patients might respond to a given treatment, and informs the selection of appropriate outcome measures to determine efficacy. He described that treatment theory tells you whether a treatment should or should not succeed at changing its "direct object," which may or may not translate into "effectiveness" in the sense of meaningfully improved function (as in the example of successfully strengthening leg muscles in two patients, one of whom has a terrible balance problem). The strengthening may only be "effective" in promoting community mobility in the patient with good balance.

In contrast, enablement theory provides no tools for change (and is indifferent to how change is made); rather, it predicts the effects that a specific intervention will have elsewhere in the ICF—that is, at levels above (see Figure 3-3) that at which the intervention was made. An important contribution of enablement theory is that it informs subject selection for effectiveness research. This is because enablement theory informs the selection of the patients in whom treatment is most likely to result in effective outcomes. In addition, it helps researchers to trace the various functions that together contribute to a higher, more complex function, and to look at whether they have treatment options for other lower-level functions that also support the desired higher-level function.

Placebos

Whyte contrasted the use of placebos in drug studies and in behavioral research, discussing how true placebos are impossible to come by in behavioral studies. A placebo must be fully plausible but guaranteed to be inert. In pharmaceutical research, in which the active ingredient is known and consists of a specific molecule, the use of a placebo allows the researcher to control for all other variables. In behavioral research it is very hard to mask the active ingredient because the interventions involve the performance of meaningful tasks. For example, patients concerned about memory generally know whether the researcher is talking about memory or something irrelevant for memory. Consequently, researchers must decide at each stage of research what confounds they are most concerned with—whether it is the natural recovery process, or patient or clinician bias—and control for them in specific ways that do not rely on placebos.

The Maturation of Research

Whyte outlined an example of a research strategy following the maturational process, highlighting where and how treatment and enablement theory play a role.

First Stage: Proof of Concept

In an early stage of research involving proof of concept, the reliance is exclusively on treatment theory. The researcher is investigating whether the essential ingredients act on the treatment object in the manner hypothesized; he or she is not yet focused on the intervention's effect on clinical outcomes. At this stage the intervention is being optimized in terms of delivery, dose, and impact, and the outcomes measured will be those most tightly tied (the most proximal) to the intervention. The researcher is developing and modifying the treatment protocol and moving it toward a manual. In terms of patient selection, the treatment theory will dictate the kinds of patients who are likely to demonstrate the most powerful and measurable impact on the treatment object under study. Even at this early stage, Whyte described how a comparison group might be called for, especially if the research is focused on the acute stage of recovery, in which rapid natural recovery is happening concurrent with the treatment. Other questions related to research design involve natural history (where are patients on the spectrum of spontaneous recovery?), and how visible are the treatment ingredients and therefore how much blinding is realistic and, if it is not, how should bias be handed?

Second Stage: Efficacy Studies

Once the initial research has shown the intervention to work as intended in a small group of patients, the next stage in the maturational process involves efficacy studies in larger groups of patients and with interventions delivered by a larger number of practitioners. These studies are still largely guided by treatment theory. At this point, the treatment becomes more formalized, and manuals and training algorithms are developed. Researchers aim to verify that the intervention affects the treatment object in a broader sample of patients and facilities, they further explore safety considerations, and they may look for early evidence of impact on clinically important outcomes in specific populations. Study participants are patients who will benefit from improvement in the treatment object as well as in some proximal clinically relevant targets. Questions in play at this stage of research design include: What are appropriate comparison treatments at this point? Does the dosage need to be adjusted or the manual changed? What are the appropriate—relatively proximal—distal outcome measures?

Third Stage: Two Types of Effectiveness Research

The third stage described by Whyte is research on the effectiveness of the intervention in routine application. He suggested dividing effectiveness research into two areas. One is by the traditional definition of effectiveness: Does the treatment have the same effect on the target when delivered by a wide range of practitioners in the field (i.e., people who may lack specialized training and practice far from academic centers of research)? This definition of effectiveness is still focused on the treatment object. The second type of effectiveness to be assessed is more rehabilitation specific, namely, the effectiveness of an intervention on distal clinical outcomes. This strand of effectiveness research relies mainly on enablement theory. It is no longer a question of whether the treatment's effects are strong enough, but rather the question is in whom can this treatment alone deliver major clinical benefit, and in whom can this treatment deliver major clinical benefit if it is provided in combination with specific other treatments?

Key questions for research design at this point include

- What kinds of patients are likely to routinely receive this treatment?
- What kinds of facilities are likely to routinely deliver it?
- Are there characteristics of patients and facilities that might moderate how effective the treatment is and that we should be measuring?

Regarding the treatment itself and optimal comparisons, it may be more relevant to compare it to the standard of care or to what is current in practice than to make a theoretically driven comparison. Regarding effectiveness, outcomes related to the object of treatment will continue to be measured, and, in addition, outcome measures will be added that are more distal and are connected to closely related targets of treatment. Research designs will need to assess overall effectiveness at the level of distal impact that is realistic. This includes evaluating patients that experience broad impact from the treatment alone as well as when the treatment is given as part of a package. If a package of treatments is given, then an algorithm is needed to decide what treatment(s) each patient receives.

Regarding this third stage, Whyte noted that it can be increasingly difficult to do randomized clinical trials, and researchers may need to rely more heavily on health services research. Whyte suggested that, as the Military Health System considers introducing certain CRT interventions, one thing it might consider is to introduce them systematically and in staggered fashion in order to produce naturalistic evidence of the effect of those interventions.

Final Remarks

Whyte recognized that not all behavioral research follows this methodical sequence. Some treatments are in wide use with little theoretical foundation. Likewise, other treatment packages are in wide use, while little is known about which specific ingredients are most important and for which patients. Some treatments are effective at the group level but differ in their effectiveness for individual people; moderating variables are in play that are poorly understood.

Whyte noted that for CRT to be rigorously shown to be effective, it will require multiple studies, and the goals of those studies will and should differ over time as the research moves through the maturational process. Using treatment theory and enablement theory in combination can guide study designs so researchers do not place unrealistic requirements on treatments while at the same time being most likely to capture the treatment benefits when they exist. He emphasized that, whether or not a research program is moving methodically through the above steps, this outline of the maturational process for CRT is useful as a reference point and for guiding researchers to regularly ask (1) Where along the path does this treatment dwell right now?, and (2) What questions need to be answered in order to move it forward?

GUIDELINES FOR CREATING MEANINGFUL DESCRIPTIONS OF CRT INTERVENTIONS

Current State of Practice

Marcel Dijkers, Senior Investigator, Brain Injury Research Center of Mount Sinai Hospital, discussed common descriptions of rehabilitation interventions, focusing on their generality and arguing for greater specificity in order to more efficiently advance a broader research agenda. Therapy descriptions of the most general type specify only the number of hours provided and the type of health care professional who provided them (e.g., 2 hours of physical therapy and 6 hours of occupational therapy). Descriptions are also often given in terms of the intended outcome (2 hours of gait therapy) or theoretical orientation (2 hours of neurodevelopmental therapy). None of these descriptions gives information about the nature, intensity, or quality of the teaching; manipulations; or instructions delivered by the therapist.

Dijkers spoke about a review that he and colleagues performed of published reports of intervention studies in which they found that the number of words used to describe the research outcomes far surpassed the words used to describe the interventions themselves. Descriptions of interventions generally covered the number of hours, the number of sessions, the discipline of the therapists, and the setting; the details of the treatments remained virtually invisible.

Dijkers cited a literature review of 95 randomized clinical trials that sought to determine the effective elements of interventions in terms of patient and treatment characteristics, treatment goals, and outcomes, with a major focus on the content of the therapy (van Heugten et al., 2012). The authors found very little information about the actual content of the treatment, either in the papers reporting on the randomized clinical trials or in other papers by the same authors.

Attempts to Classify Rehabilitation Treatments

Dijkers explored several possible schemes for categorizing rehabilitation interventions. One option, medical subject headings, are useful for locating published work, but as descriptions for rehabilitation interventions they leave much to be desired. The category of "therapeutics" has a subcategory of rehabilitation, but the associated terms are very general and in some cases overlapping. The classification system of the International Classification of Functioning Disability and Health has *health services* and *health systems* as subcategories of *environment*. Although CRT and rehabilitation are contained within these descriptions, the system lacks the specificity necessary to be useful. The ICF also characterizes patients' treatments based on the targeted outcome. However, this also says nothing about what the intervention entailed. Even when the target constitutes the treatment, for example, in gait therapy in which the gait is improved by the patient's practicing an improved gait, simply naming the target provides little useful information about the actual intervention.

An attempt was made within practice-based evidence studies funded by the National Institute on Disability and Rehabilitation Research to compile lists of names given to interventions based on discussions among treatment providers. Providers supplied sets of names for the treatments they used that were expected to have an impact on patient outcomes. For TBI, lists of activities and interventions were drawn up, divided by type (e.g., physical therapy and psychology). But in neither case were the terms specific enough to shed any light on what the intervention consisted of.

Dijkers discussed treatment typologies in health care, including Current Procedural Terminology (CPT) and Systematized Nomenclature of Medicine (SNOMED). He found Current Procedural Terminology problematic for CRT-related terms because it sometimes gathered together interventions under one code that warranted separate codes and, conversely, it sometimes split multiple interventions among different codes when they ought to have shared just one. SNOMED's terminology system suffered from similar issues. The nursing intervention classification system goes into greater detail with regard to interventions, each one of which is labeled, defined, and described using from 1 to 20 specific nursing activities. This system includes an array of activities and interventions specific to TBI, approaching usefulness much more closely than do the previous classification schemes. However, this system remains too general to contribute much to the advancement of research on CRT for TBI.

More Promising Ways of Describing Rehabilitation Treatment

Dijkers turned to what he and others view as essential components of a framework that will allow researchers studying CRT for TBI to fruitfully describe, study, and communicate about their work. This framework was the same as that described earlier by John Whyte and centered on specifying essential ingredients, those attributes of the treatment that bring about changes in the object of treatment (and that often are the basis for naming the treatment) through a hypothesized mechanism of action. The changes in the object of treatment may cascade to more distal outcomes in the treatment target. Dijkers highlighted the usefulness of separating (proximal) objects of treatment from (distal, higher-level) targets of treatment, noting how a single treatment target (e.g., the patient dressing him- or herself) may be addressed by multiple means, through different objects of treatment.

When classifying interventions, while researchers often think in terms of ingredients (and mechanisms), practitioners think first in terms of objects (and targets) of treatment—what problem does the patient have, and how can it be improved? Dijkers suggested that rather than classifying interventions by the ingredients, researchers might consider classifying them first by the object and then using subcategories consisting of different sets of ingredients.

Content of Interventions and Dose

Dijkers discussed dose and dosage as a way to think through important issues concerning active ingredients. In the pharmacological model that informs the current notion of dosage, the active ingredient is a molecule and dosage is defined in terms of quantity of the molecules given per certain characteristics of the patient—body weight, severity of disease or disorder, and so on. However, to apply the notion of *dosage* to CRT raises a number of questions that have not yet been investigated. Is any dose of CRT beneficial? Is there an optimal amount or intensity of CRT? When does CRT end, and how do we decide?

Dijkers offered the example of a CRT intervention at his institution, the Brain Injury Research Center of Mount Sinai Hospital, highlighting the concept of an active ingredient in action. His research team has a program providing remediation of executive function, attention training, and emotional regulation. A key element of the program is a strategy they have termed "SWAPS":

- Stop.
- What is the problem?
- Alternatives?
- Pick one and plan.
- Satisfied?

When a patient is faced with a problem, he or she applies SWAPS, and Dijkers proposed that SWAPS is the active ingredient. To sharpen the definition of this CRT intervention, Dijkers drew on work by Steven Page's research group that proposed "intensity," "dosing," and "delivery method" as key elements of stroke motor rehabilitation (Page et al., 2012). Dijkers also highlighted a set of papers recently published in the *International Journal of Speech and Language Pathology* on optimal treatment intensity (motivated by the question of the appropriate point at which to discharge a patient). One paper defined "treatment intensity" as the number of repetitions of an active ingredient delivered during a treatment session and discussed optimal treatment intensities. It was followed by journal-solicited comments and critiques from practitioners in a variety of fields, and then by a second paper by the original authors describing how they saw the state of the field and discussing why establishing the optimal intensity of an intervention is difficult (Baker, 2012). Dijkers recommended these papers as examples of sound thinking on the questions of dosage, but noted that the authors had not begun to think in terms of active ingredients and how to quantify, measure, and operationalize them—indicating that even they had a long way to go before arriving at a research design capable of constituting a solid step along the translational pipeline. To date, there have been no studies that have elucidated the effective dose needed to achieve a given outcome at the termination of treatment and whether this dose needs to be altered if desired effects are to be maintained over time.

4

Key Themes

After the three opening presentations set the stage for discussion, the workshop participants were divided into small groups and asked to analyze three published research papers on cognitive rehabilitation therapy (CRT) for traumatic brain injury (TBI). Workshop participants had been provided with the three papers and a list of questions for each prior to the workshop. Committee members had drafted the discussion questions, and a committee member moderated each small-group discussion. The discussion of the three papers was not intended to reassess the papers' conclusions; rather, the discussions were designed to elicit participants' suggestions about the elements of optimal research design and the succession of studies through the maturational process. Participants evaluated variables such as sample size, patient selection, description of interventions, and selection and measurement of outcomes, with an eye toward generalizing their assessments to inform the design of future studies. Following each small-group discussion, a member of each group reported back to the entire group and a free-ranging discussion ensued. This chapter summarizes the key themes in the report-back sessions. As was noted in Chapter 1, all ideas and suggestions expressed by participants do not reflect a consensus and should not be interpreted as such.

THE TRANSLATIONAL PIPELINE AND RESEARCH DESIGN

Balancing Urgency vs. Evidence

Health service administrators and service providers must choose which interventions to pursue by balancing competing needs: the magnitude of patients' needs, the magnitude of the intervention's benefit, the cost of the research, and the cost of the intervention itself. There was a good deal of discussion about the continuum from "implement something immediately" to "wait and research interventions thoroughly." Participants explored the question, how clear does the evidence need to be for an intervention to be worth implementing? At one end of the continuum is the decision to implement interventions right away (without as strong of evidence of efficacy as might be desired) and to plan subsequent research based on what the implementation showed. At the other end of the continuum is the decision to more rigorously determine which interventions are effective and why, followed then by implementation. Individual participants expressed favor for each strategy, depending on the balance of urgency, the effect size, cost-effectiveness, and other factors.

Promoting Continuity in the Research Pipeline

Several participants agreed on the need for greater continuity in the translational pipeline for using CRT to treat TBI. For any given domain (attention, executive function, language and social communication, visuospatial perception, and memory) and patient population (severity of injury, stage of recovery), there are few published papers that describe in detail what the intervention was, what kind of feedback was measured, and what the schedule of feedback was—the dynamic process for behavioral intervention. The problem is rooted in the structure of research cultures in which researchers are often very siloed—a single researcher or team does not have expertise along the entire translational pipeline, from idea generation to proof of concept to broad implementation. This section of the summary highlights the overarching points raised about study design and addresses the challenges of creating and maintaining a research pipeline that has the necessary continuity between research approaches as a research program moves through the maturational process discussed by John Whyte and summarized in Chapter 3.

Organization and Pace of the Maturational Process

Individual participants offered several bird's-eye perspectives on research design. These options were tailored to the challenge of addressing complex health problems with a complex set of interventions, as is the case for using CRT for TBI.

Dismantling vs. Additive

A "dismantling" approach begins with a large, complex problem and works with the individual components of intervention to determine which ones are essential. An "additive" approach, in contrast, begins with the individual components known to be effective and then combines them in a package. The additive approach requires that small improvements from focused interventions be accepted as progress; they may later be combined into a program that includes an algorithm to determine which components are provided to a given patient.

Using Dismantling and Additive Approaches Simultaneously

Several participants were in favor of doing top-down and bottom-up research simultaneously, a view held usually in an effort to balance urgency with building an evidence base.

In addition, one participant brought up the idea of adopting the venture capital model of disruptive innovation, suggesting that the research community may want to consider a nonlinear approach to the complex problem of using CRT for TBI. A model of disruptive innovation could be put to work to search for the one-in-a-million intervention that changes the paradigm and profoundly alters the standard of care; it could be combined with a model of incremental improvement.[1]

When to Optimize?

Looking more closely at the movement of a research program along the maturational process, participants examined the question of when a nascent study is ready to be optimized. They explored the question faced by researchers—at the conclusion of a study—of whether to move forward in the maturational process (toward larger studies) or to continue examining the intervention to try to increase the effect size and determine what the active ingredients are. When researchers choose the former, it means investigating whether an intervention that works in one place also works more broadly (more patients, more facilities), and this requires freezing

---

[1] "Disruptive innovation" is a concept used in the business world, referring to new companies entering new markets with a lower-priced product related to higher-priced products in more lucrative markets. The application of this concept to health care research may revolve around seeing treatments as either new markets or new products—the possibility of trying many low-cost, unconventional interventions in an attempt to stumble somewhat blindly onto the desired combination of inexpensive and effective.

the intervention and studying it in broader populations and delivered by more practitioners. When researchers opt for the latter, it means spending more time ensuring that the intervention warrants broader testing, increasing its impact on patient health, and determining which of the ingredients are delivering the effect and whether different ingredients deliver different elements of it.

The considerations underlying this choice are both scientific and pragmatic. One scientific consideration is the effect size. If the effect size is very large (or just significant and the intervention is inexpensive), researchers may opt to take it to the next point in the maturational process. If the effect size is only borderline and the intervention is costly, this might indicate the wisdom of improving the intervention's impact before proceeding. In many cases, both forces are acting on the decision (the need to have an implementable intervention and the need for more data on a promising one), and the question becomes one of priority and resources.

Pragmatic concerns include the cost of the research and of the intervention itself and how cost compares to the magnitude of the effect and the level of need among the patient population. If an intervention is very expensive, the researcher may be satisfied with the effect size but may want to increase the impact so the intervention can be delivered, for example, less frequently or more quickly. If the intervention is relatively inexpensive and relatively effective, the researcher may choose to optimize it immediately.

SEVERITY LEVELS OF TBI: DISCUSSION OF MILD INJURY

Workshop participants individually offered suggestions and ideas concerning the needs specific to mild TBI, the form of TBI affecting the largest number of military personnel.

Definitions and Distinctions

Mild, Moderate, and Severe

A participant raised the question of how the current classification of mild, moderate, and severe may affect research outcomes. Others raised the question using a typology of symptoms to characterize people rather than the current classification system. One participant expressed the opinion that the definition of mild brain injury is the weakest part of the research agenda and that it limits the research community's ability to make progress in the treatment of TBI.

Distinction Between Mild TBI from Which an Individual Recovers and Mild TBI That Leads to Chronic Symptoms

Another participant spoke about the distinction between mild injuries from which a person recovers quickly and mild injuries that are followed by chronic complaints and a longer presentation of symptoms. She encouraged the group not to think of these two as existing along a definite continuum but rather as discrete situations. She discussed how when military service members suffer mild TBIs in combat, often the more quickly they receive interventions to mitigate the damage of the injury and see an expectation of recovery, the more likely they are to be able to return to duty within a short time. Therefore, it is desirable to have early models of intervention to prevent long-term effects, including a "disabled mentality." She noted that a second factor affecting whether an injury will become chronic is an individual's comorbidities. Thus, given that not all mild brain injuries have serious, long-term consequences, and given that it is possible that some multipronged interventions could make an individual's condition worse, she believed that it is important to develop a prognostic framework for mild TBI including the role played by comorbidities.

The Origins of the Functional Deficit, and Keeping It Distinct from a Cognitive Impairment

One participant cautioned against assuming that the cause of a cognitive difficulty is a cognitive impairment. She highlighted that a practitioner treating a person with a brain injury is not necessarily treating the brain injury per se, but is treating the cognitive deficit. The deficit may be caused by factors other than an actual cognitive impairment—for example, pain. Also emphasized was the distinction between symptoms (regardless of etiology) and a documented deficit, and the importance for a given study of an intervention of determining whether or not symptoms and deficits need to be teased apart.

Closing the Knowledge Gap

The participants discussed the development of an action plan for mild TBI that would close the many gaps identified in the Institute of Medicine (IOM) report *Cognitive Rehabilitation Therapy for Traumatic Brain Injury: Evaluating the Evidence*. Such an action plan might fall on the "immediate" end of the spectrum since the clinical need is so great. One participant suggested that the research community may have been unduly distracted by the severe clinical needs of patients with moderate-to-severe TBI, to the detriment of research on mild injuries, which are much more common. He suggested that the research community consider beginning with the patients with milder injuries, learn how to develop effective treatments, and extrapolate to treating patients with more severe deficits.[2]

Several participants discussed how studies of interventions that have low-grade (but very important) effects will need to be very large and the intervention will need to have a strong impact, if the signal is to be separated from the "noise" of natural recovery. One participant recommended a grassroots approach to arriving at initial standardization (manualization). Since mild TBI is associated with a combination of issues (e.g., sensory, cognitive, and psychological problems, and symptoms such as fatigue and pain), it may be undesirable to separate out cognitive impairment too early. It can be difficult to compile a complete picture of the condition of someone with mild TBI unless comorbidities and environmental factors are taken into account. One option would be to solicit clinical impressions of effectiveness (from patient accounts and standardized measures), particularly around areas of transition in recovery, and then attempt to standardize and manualize the interventions—still in multi-ingredient form—and test them on a broader scale. (This constitutes an examples of the "dismantling" approach discussed earlier.)

COMPONENTS OF RESEARCH STUDIES AND THEIR CHARACTERISTICS AT DIFFERENT POINTS IN THE MATURATIONAL PROCESS

Below is a thematic summary of suggestions offered by individual workshop participants in either the reporting-back sessions following small-group discussions or in discussions after the formal presentations. All suggestions originated with one or several participants, and no views expressed here represent a consensus.

Treatment Theory and Enablement Theory

It is important that a specific treatment theory be articulated in a research report, raising questions of active and essential ingredients and the mechanism of action, all of which help the study to provide a stronger basis for future studies that build on it.

---

[2] Interventions for mild TBI may not always generalize to moderate and severe TBI, and this should be considered in study design and interpretation.

Study Design

Different types of questions lend themselves to different types of analysis. One participant noted that when the target of treatment is at the activity and participation level, and when the intervention is very broadly based, a health services implementation approach might be optimal. In contrast, a very focused intervention, such as attention process training, would be a good candidate for a more traditional, classical research design. Individual participants posited the following suggestions:

- Pre-post or single-subject designs are useful.
- Mixed methods—qualitative/quantitative—can be useful.
- Observational studies could be used more commonly as an initial phase of research.
- To test specific active ingredients, a design that is tighter than observational would be needed.
- Factorial designs could be considered to compare treatment packages in order to gain power with a smaller sample size (as long as there are no adverse effects between the interventions).

Regarding studies of compensatory strategies specifically, individual participants noted the need to separately evaluate the acquisition of the strategy and the impact of using the strategy on the target domain. One participant noted how in some cases the strategies can be commercializable products. Thinking of them as products can be beneficial because it obligates the researcher to test not only efficacy but also usability and acceptability, and to think about how the product is presented—for example, on a card, a notebook, or a smartphone application. Having commercializable products also opens up new funding streams, such as Small Business Innovation Research and Small Business Technology Transfer grants.

Overall, individual participants suggested the following study design elements as the most useful or advantageous:

- Outcomes that are meaningful to the patient
- Interventions that are or could be manualizable
- Designs that are flexible and expandable across populations (e.g., severity of injury)
- Relatively short studies that are not resource intensive and are easily built upon
- Designs with easy application to military settings (e.g., goal-management training)
- Interventions that are easily adapted to other settings

For early-stage research, some participants suggested that case reports and small studies can be valuable. They are inexpensive and can potentially detect a "signal" that subsequent studies can follow up on. Even though the focus of an early study is on impairment-level function and proximal outcomes, it is important to consider generalizability as well—tracking whether improving impairment-level function has any effect on even slightly more general functions.

For mid-stage research, participants suggested that adaptive types of designs be considered to obtain information in real time and alter an arm of a randomized clinical trial. They proposed that factorial designs be considered to compare treatment packages and thus gain power with smaller sample sizes (as long as there are not any adverse effects between the interventions). To simultaneously change the study design and broaden the population, a research team could either carry out a randomized clinical trial with three arms or do two sequential studies. The trial would have a control (standard of care) and two variables, each of which could be compared to the standard of care and to one another.

For late-stage and multisite research, individual workshop participants proposed that adaptive types of designs be considered to obtain information in real time and alter an arm of a randomized clinical trial and that factorial designs be considered to compare treatment packages and thus gain power with smaller sample sizes (as long as there are not any adverse effects between the interventions). They discussed that delayed-start designs, in which two randomized groups start in a staggered fashion, can also be beneficial. At this late stage of effectiveness research, it may be increasingly difficult to do randomized clinical trials. It may be necessary to rely more heavily on health services research, and as the Military Health System considers introducing procedures or programs, one thing they could consider is introducing them systematically and in staggered fashion such that we get naturalistic evidence of the impact of those introductions. For large-scale studies to yield key information, an essential component is a set of outcome measures that are robust, sensitive, and easily implemented in the field. Multisite networks have an advantage for heterogeneous populations in which patients often have difficulty participating (e.g., transportation to site). Multisite networks make it possible to optimize the power of the network; they also encourage standardization and generalizability of results. If a study is being done at multiple sites, it needs a measure of the quality of treatment provision, that is, the delivery of ingredients (which requires us to define the ingredients that must be delivered). A protocolized manual is required.

Patient Inclusion/Exclusion

Discussion among the participants denoted that it is important to characterize the specific deficits of patients, their social support systems, and covariates (e.g., education, intact memory). Participants identified the several advantages of heterogeneity or homogeneity of the patient population at different points in the maturational process. For early- to mid-stage research, it can be beneficial for a follow-up study to use a more heterogeneous sample, one that includes comorbidities different than those in the earlier study. After a small heterogeneous study, it can also be beneficial to move to a more homogeneous group for variables such as diagnosis, severity level, type of injury, and age. To ensure that a study uses a representative patient population that could still plausibly benefit from the intervention, it may be necessary to broaden the heterogeneity of the patient population. Recruitment efforts should be diversified in order to include patients other than those referred by physicians. Finally, it is important to match the patient characteristics to the outcome(s) being evaluated (i.e., who the intervention is good for, and at what point in time will they benefit from it?).

Interventions

Individual participants remarked that it is important that an intervention be *delivered uniformly* and that the study design ensures that uniform delivery take place. For interventions with multiple components, it is important to determine which component contains the *essential ingredient*. For interventions to have the desired effect, there must not be preconditions that prevent the effect (other impairments than the one under study). If there are preconditions, then additional interventions might be necessary to address them as well. If a study is being conducted at multiple sites, it needs a measure of the quality of treatment provision—delivery of ingredients (which requires us to define the ingredients that must be delivered in a protocolized manual). Flexible interventions are advantageous in early studies as a basic approach; if researchers see a benefit in one patient population and go on to study different populations, they will be able to implement a flexible intervention relatively easily. Finally, "treatments" discussed in a paper are often technically *more than one treatment*. For example, when a treatment is compensatory, there are two components: the selection of the device and the use of the device. The success of either of these components is dependent on several variables having to do with the practitioner, the patient, and the treatment.

Targets

Impairment-based research is more straightforward (researchers can make inferences more directly) than research on a broader disability. Workshop participants pointed out that it is important to target an *impairment* as opposed to a *task* or an entire domain. Interventions that target a task are less than ideal because they do not lend themselves to generalization. Interventions that target a domain (e.g., executive function) are less than ideal because they are so broad as to make it difficult to describe outcomes. Therefore, it is preferable that interventions target a specific functional impairment. Such functionally based interventions are generally more useful than interventions that "train to the outcome."

Studies in which the target is a very focused impairment-level problem may lend themselves to a randomized clinical trial much more easily than studies in which the target is broadly based. For studies in which the target is very broad, researchers could consider an implementation-style research program in which the intervention is rolled out and its effects looked at broadly. Simultaneously, the effect of the components of the broad study could be examined more specifically.

Outcomes

Select participants highlighted the importance of measuring and having data on *patient-centered outcomes*. The IOM report *Cognitive Rehabilitation Therapy for Traumatic Brain Injury: Evaluating the Evidence* found a relative paucity of research on patient-centered outcomes. Although such research is not expected before efficacy has been established, it is important thereafter. As research moves through the maturational process, research on patient-centered outcomes becomes increasingly important. Consequently, it is important to do the following:

- Test the durability of effects, use proximal outcomes.
- Identify premorbid factors that might influence people's initial ability to perform a task (such as set a goal).
- Assess the ecological validity of the outcomes—the real-world impact.
- Include performance-based measures.

Regarding outcome measures using patient reporting vs. objective measures, some studies use one and would benefit from the other. Participants noted that it is important to rate outcomes to the people who matter, (e.g., patients, caregivers, family members). It is important to not alter the outcomes being assessed when a research program moves from testing efficacy to testing effectiveness.

The participants also discussed the issue of how many outcomes are appropriate to test at the same time. Some participants thought that testing multiple outcomes is best, as they can reflect different parts of the spectrum from proximal to distal. Other participants wondered whether it were possible for a single study to have too many outcomes, and whether it might be better to limit outcomes to just one. One group discussed whether it might be best to have multiple outcomes in the early stages of research, which are honed down as research progresses, or whether it is optimal to be specific and selective at the beginning, followed by a broadening of outcomes. The further a study is from having a one-to-one correspondence between intervention and target, the greater the importance of looking either for patients who have only one problem or for packages of treatments that address the multiple problems of a patient, of which attention (or one of the other domains) is just one of the patient's problems.

Controls

Participants discussed the importance of establishing control groups based on the treatment theory and its mechanism of action. Because rehabilitation involves helping people who are suffering and researchers do not want to give a patient nothing, they often do the following (which yields little useful information): A intervention and B intervention are compared, B shows no difference in effect from A, and it is thus not possible to know whether both are effective or neither is. Participants acknowledged that identifying an appropriate control can be difficult, for example, controlling for social interaction when the treatment is for social interaction. Consequently, it may sometimes be best to control for standard of care, unless very few people receive it. However, having standard of care as the control does make recruitment very difficult; therefore, wait list controls may offer a potentially better alternative.

Manuals

Workshop participants identified the great need for the protocols and manuals necessary as a starting point to further investigate specific interventions for specific patient populations and to examine interventions' cost-effectiveness. The American Congress of Rehabilitation Medicine has published a cognitive rehabilitation training manual, which at this time is not specific enough to guide a practitioner's treatment of a specific individual. For early, single-center studies, a fully developed manual is likely not warranted. Rather, a more "lightweight" manual could be used that guides the research team. The team may improve on it somewhat, but expending concentrated energy on the manual would wait until multicenter trials are being planned. To start an investigation, the standard of care could be manualized and then tested. One participant cautioned, however, about the possible negative effect on compliance of giving practitioners a manual, sending them out to do the treatments, and then revising from there.

DATABASES

Individual participants noted there are databases or repositories that exist or that are in the process of formation that may be useful as (1) potential sources of data, (2) may be repositories to which research could contribute, and (3) may assist researchers as they design studies and interpret findings. The National Institute on Disability and Rehabilitation Research TBI Model System's National Database is available to the public. Deidentified data are provided to outside researchers who have an interest, and researchers often have the opportunity to collaborate with those who have contributed data to the TBI Model System Centers themselves. The National Institute on Disability and Rehabilitation Research has interagency agreements with the Centers for Disease Control and Prevention and other federal agencies for the use of the database to answer key research questions, which will allow for national estimates on outcomes for diverse interventions.

In parallel with the aforementioned database, the Department of Veterans Affairs has established a database that tracks people with TBI who have been admitted for inpatient rehabilitation to four of its polytrauma rehabilitation centers. This database collects all of the same data as in the TBI Model System's National Database, as well as additional data. It will be possible, at a future date, to do comparative research across the two databases. The Common Data Element project is a collaboration among the Department of Veterans Affairs, Department of Defense, National Institutes of Health, Centers for Disease Control and Prevention, and National Institute on Disability and Rehabilitation Research. The project collects data on patient characteristics, treatments, and outcomes. Its main strength at this point is for acute care. A participant recommended that efforts coming out of this workshop build on this project. An international conversation has been going on for two to three years about the possibility of collecting high-quality, granular data across centers that would embrace the complexity of CRT for TBI—specifically for the acute stage. Such an effort would support comparative effectiveness research, allowing researchers to tease apart questions about who certain interventions work for, what treatments seem to be most effective, and the role of comorbidities.

WHO OWNS THIS PROCESS GOING FORWARD?

At several points during the workshop, individual participants expressed their appreciation for the points raised, and they asked about the next steps toward having the ideas acted upon. Who owns the new understanding of the gaps in knowledge, who will formulate an action plan, and who will set forth the expectation that the action plan be carried out? Various participants expressed the view that the process is owned by multiple stakeholders, including military and other federal government agencies, and civilian researchers. Participants noted that the question of "who" looks different when referring to the military system versus the civilian world of health care. Regarding the Military Health System, John Davison[3] noted that the military health and research units are many and dispersed, and it was his hope that the framework and suggestions laid out in the workshop would propel a continued dialogue—not only within the Department of Defense, but also among the Department of Defense, the Department of Veterans Affairs, and subject-matter experts—about the research necessary to move forward the use of CRT for TBI.

A participant noted what he considered to be an advantage had by the Military Health System, namely, that the standardization of care may be more feasible there than in the civilian sector. He expressed the opinion that the military system could be better able to establish standardized treatments, and this standardization could serve as a baseline that researchers improve upon. Another participant echoed these sentiments, mentioning the numerous sites operated by the Defense and Veterans Brain Injury Center (DVBIC), the Department of Veterans Affairs, and the planned satellites of the National Intrepid Center of Excellence as fertile ground for the manualized application of CRT interventions for TBI. In later stages of the maturational process of research on CRT for TBI, it may be necessary to rely more heavily on health services research. As the Military Health System considers introducing CRT interventions, one strategy it may want to consider is introducing CRT interventions systematically and in staggered fashion, thus obtaining naturalistic evidence of the impact of those introductions. A tempering viewpoint, however, was offered by Davison in his closing remarks, as he noted that military health care organizations experience much the same fragmentation as do civilian ones.

The role of funding agencies was raised multiple times over the course of the workshop. Some participants spoke of elements of a misalignment between what funders tend to fund and what researchers need funding for in order to methodically move research along the translational pipeline.

---

[3] Acting Director, TRICARE Management Activity/Office of the Chief Medical Officer, Behavioral Medicine Division.

Studies essential for the research maturational process include proof-of-concept studies, then efficacy studies, and ultimately effectiveness research; however, some in the group expressed concern that proof-of-concept studies were difficult to fund. One participant mentioned a discrepancy that sometimes exists between researchers' and grant review panels' views on control groups; namely, even if a research design, in order to be scientifically rigorous, calls for a control group that receives no treatment, researchers hesitate to present such a design in grant applications. At the conclusion of the workshop, John Whyte led a discussion in which he outlined three broad research strategies that could guide research decisions and help decision makers balance urgency, evidence, and cost-effectiveness.

Immediate Implementation

One strategy that the military could consider would be to take a manualized treatment shown to have significant effects in patients' daily lives, implement it, and fund studies to elucidate the active and essential ingredients and mechanism of action. If the decision were made to implement CRT interventions immediately even while the evidence supporting their effectiveness was less than solid (i.e., only moderate amounts of evidence exist), what would this mean?

Careful Selection of the Intervention

The intervention would be selected based on a carefully considered combination of existing evidence and clinical importance. Factors to be weighed would include the magnitude and importance of the problem—how many members of the military suffer from it? One might opt against implementing an intervention with somewhat stronger evidence but that addresses a problem that few patients have, in favor of implementing an intervention that has weaker evidence but that addresses a very common problem.

Standardization of the Intervention

The intervention would need to be standardized and operationalized even if it were still unknown whether the treatment was effective; it would be crucial that researchers precisely define that which they are studying. The committee charged with the original IOM report found it difficult to determine what a given intervention consisted of; therefore, more complete, precise definitions going forward will greatly support forward movement toward fuller knowledge of different interventions. Manualization would allow researchers to assess consistency of delivery (e.g., same name of intervention, same services, same billing code), as well as systematically manipulate different elements of the intervention over time.

One advantage of this approach, in practical terms, would be that if a researcher is able to demonstrate a practical benefit from an intervention, he or she may be better able to secure funding for subsequent studies focused on the nuances of the intervention—the mechanism of action and active and essential ingredients. Another potential advantage is that it may not only advance knowledge about a specific intervention but could also foster a climate of forward movement for CRT for TBI overall.

A Middle Way: A Quasi-Experimental Health Services Design Component

A second strategy described by Whyte was a middle road, a path that beckoned somewhat less to the immediate need to implement interventions and leaned more toward establishing more robust evidence for an intervention's effectiveness.

Selection of the Intervention

In this case the intervention would be selected based also on a combination of existing evidence and the research target's clinical importance, in this instance putting somewhat more weight on the desirability of empirical evidence supporting an intervention's effectiveness. The intervention would be standardized and operationalized as described above.

Experimental Design

One consideration for research design would be to assess what outcome measures are optimal to reveal the effects of the intervention. The level of function of the outcome would need to be measured carefully. For example, to measure a high-level outcome, such as returning to work, it would not be appropriate for an intervention to address a specific impairment (such as a memory problem) that is only one of many impairments associated with the high-level outcome.

The intervention might be implemented in a staggered fashion, which would allow researchers to see whether the phasing of impact matches the phasing of implementation.

It would be important to ensure that what is being measured were the results of the treatment's implementation, and not patient variation.

A Research-Heavy, Conservative Approach

A third strategy would lean most strongly in favor of rigorously establishing the effectiveness of an intervention and moving conceptually sound and promising treatments along the translational pipeline. Such an approach might involve the following:

- Carry out smaller maturational studies aimed specifically at gaining more evidence for effectiveness—identify the active and essential ingredients.
- Pay explicit attention to treatment ingredients, attempts to operationalize them, and attempts to measure their delivery.
- Implement interventions as the evidence mounts.
- Continue with quasi-experimental health services research to investigate "routine delivery," because the evidence would have been obtained in controlled conditions and the intervention would then need to be used by a variety of practitioners in a variety of institutions and settings.

CLOSING REMARKS

John Whyte urged all participants—researchers and health services administrators in the civilian and military worlds—to continue considering what directions they think will be most productive, where resources should be directed, and what the opportunities are, given whom they treat and for what health concerns. What elements of common research strategies have hindered clear progress toward solid evidence in favor of specific CRTs? What research strategies promise to increase momentum? As the Military Health System considers implementing interventions that hold the promise of improving patients' lives, where should it focus, and why?

The question for health services administrators and practitioners of CRT, in Whyte's view, comes down to finding an optimal way to make decisions—the published evidence is not strong enough to guide decisions singlehandedly. Decision makers will need to sort through the pros and cons of the early implementation of treatments versus continued, more formal research, given variables such as the range of evidence and the prevalence and severity of the problem, the cost of interventions, and the cost of the research.

John Davison offered his thanks to the workshop participants, saying that the workshop had been very instructive for himself and his colleagues from TRICARE, and he expressed the hope that the dialogue would continue. He drew parallels between the process of arriving at manualized treatment for post-traumatic stress disorder (PTSD), which has been accomplished, and the process of arriving at manualized treatment for TBI, which is still very much under way. In the case of PTSD, he noted how external pressure had been important for moving the process forward; the Military Health System benefitted from outside voices asking why they were not using the most evidence-based approaches.

Addressing a question that came up several times during the workshop—that of who owns this process of advancing the state of the field—Davison acknowledged that just as researchers have a diversity of interests and concerns, so do the various branches of the organizations concerned with TBI among military service members. Centers of Excellence, research offices, clinical proponency offices, and others are "all touching different parts of the elephant." He related the need expressed by leaders of the military health research program, namely, clinical practice guidelines for using CRT to treat TBI. In concrete terms, he noted how the original IOM report and the current workshop will be of great help to TRICARE and the Department of Defense as it makes more informed, focused program announcements in the future on CRT research directions. Finally, Davison reiterated the commitment of TRICARE to helping service members who suffer from TBIs of any type, and he asserted that the responsibility is on TRICARE's systems to better coordinate efforts and, ultimately, arrive at clinical guidelines for using CRT to treat TBI in a way that is effective, evidence-based, and the most efficient use of dollars possible.

References

Baker, E. 2012. Optimal intervention intensity in speech-language pathology: Discoveries, challenges, and unchartered territories. *International Journal of Speech-Language Pathology* 14(5):478-485.

DVBIC (Defense and Veterans Brain Injury Center). 2011. *DoD worldwide numbers for TBI: Total diagnoses*. http://www.dvbic.org/dod-worldwide-numbers-tbi (accessed November 6, 2012).

Harley, J. P., C. Allen, T. L. Braciszewski, K. D. Cicerone, C. Dahlberg, S. Evans, M. Foto, W. A. Gordon, D. Harrington, W. Levin, J. F. Malec, S. Millis, J. Morris, C. Muir, J. Richert, E. Salazar, D. A. Schiavone, and J. S. Smigelski. 1992. Guidelines for cognitive rehabilitation. *NeuroRehabilitation* 2(3):62-67.

Page, S. J., A. Schmid, and J. E. Harris. 2012. Optimizing terminology for stroke motor rehabilitation: Recommendations from the American Congress of Rehabilitation Medicine Stroke Movement Interventions Subcommittee. *Archives of Physical Medicine and Rehabilitation* 93(8):1395-1399.

Snell, F. I., and M. J. Halter. 2010. A signature wound of war. *Journal of Psychosocial Nursing and Mental Health Services* 48(2):22-28.

van Heugten, C., G. Wolters Gregório, and D. Wade. 2012. Evidence-based cognitive rehabilitation after acquired brain injury: A systematic review of content of treatment. *Neuropsychological Rehabilitation* 22(5):653-673.

Appendix A

Recommendations of the IOM Report *Cognitive Rehabilitation Therapy for Traumatic Brain Injury: Evaluating the Evidence*

Considering the dearth of conclusive evidence identified to date, the committee recommends an investment in research to further develop cognitive rehabilitation therapy (CRT). [. . .] The evidence provides limited, and in some cases modest, support for the efficacy of CRT interventions. However, the limitations of the evidence do not rule out meaningful benefit. The committee defined *limited* evidence as "Interpretable results from a single study or mixed results from two or more studies" and *modest* evidence as "Two or more studies reporting interpretable, informative, and largely similar results" [. . .]. **The committee emphasizes that conclusions based on the limited evidence regarding the effectiveness of CRT does not indicate that the effectiveness of CRT treatments are "limited;" the limitations of the evidence do not rule out meaningful benefit.** *In fact, the committee supports the ongoing clinical application of CRT interventions for individuals with cognitive and behavioral deficits due to traumatic brain injury (TBI).* One way policy could reflect the provision of CRT is to facilitate the application of best-supported techniques in TBI patients in the chronic phase (where natural recovery is less of a confound), with the proviso that objectively measurable functional goals are articulated and tracked and that treatment continues only so long as gains are noted.

To acquire more specific, meaningful results from future research the committee has laid out a comprehensive research agenda to overcome challenges in determining efficacy and effectiveness. These recommendations are therefore possible because the evidence review signals some promise. However, to improve future evaluations of efficacy and effectiveness of CRT for TBI, larger sample sizes and volume of data are required, particularly to answer questions about which patients benefit most from which treatment(s). This requires more extensive funding of experimental trials and a commitment to mining clinical practice data in the most rigorous way possible. For such approaches to be most informative, the variables that characterize patient heterogeneity, the outcomes that are used to measure impact of treatment, and the treatments themselves need to be defined and standardized. In addition, more rigorous review of potential harm or adverse events related to specific CRT treatments is necessary.

Nascent efforts at standardization are under way across multiple civilian and military funding agencies. These efforts should take place in collaboration. The National Institutes of Health (NIH) common data element (CDE) initiative, a National Institute on Disability and Rehabilitation Research (NIDRR)-supported center on treatment definition, and several practice-based evidence studies are helping to better characterize TBI patients, treatments, and relevant outcomes. Practice-based evidence studies include the Congressionally Mandated Longitudinal Study on TBI, DVBIC Study on Cognitive Rehabilitation Effectiveness for Mild TBI (SCORE!), Millennium, and TBI Model Systems. These cohorts involve collaborative efforts between the Department of Defense (DoD) and the Veterans Administration (VA) via the Defense and Veterans Brain Injury Center (DVBIC). The committee recognizes the ongoing emphasis from both government agencies to enhance collaboration for TBI and psychological health of service members and veterans through the VA/DoD Joint Executive Council Strategic Plan to integrate health care services. [. . .] This collaboration is especially important in evaluating and maintaining transitions in care and long-term treatment for injured soldiers as they move out of the Military Health System (MHS) and into the VA's health care system, the Veterans Health System.

Because CRT is not a single therapy, questions of efficacy and effectiveness need to be answered for each cognitive domain and by treatment approach. Nevertheless, within a specific cognitive domain, there must be sufficient research and replication for conclusions to be drawn. Standard definitions for intervention type, content, and key ingredients will be critical to developing evidence-based practice standards. The documentation of interventions in practice and more frequent use of manual-based interventions in research will help validate measures of treatment fidelity. For example, while there is evidence from controlled trials that internal memory strategies are useful for improving recall on decontextualized, standard tests of memory, there is limited evidence that these benefits translate into meaningful changes in patients' everyday memory either for specific tasks/activities or for avoiding memory failures. Therefore, an increased emphasis on functional patient-centered outcomes would allow for a more meaningful translation from cognitive domain to patient functioning.

The committee recommends the DoD undertake the following:

Recommendation 14-1: The DoD should work with other rehabilitation research and funding organizations to:
1. Identify and select uniform data elements characterizing TBI patients including cognitive impairments (to supplement measures of injury severity) and key premorbid conditions, comorbidities, and environmental factors that may influence recovery and treatment response;
2. Identify and select uniform TBI outcome measures, including standard measures of cognitive and global/functional outcomes; and
3. Create a plan of action to:
   a. Identify currently feasible methods of measuring the delivery of CRT interventions;
   b. Advance the development of a taxonomy for CRT interventions that can be used for this purpose in the future; and
   c. Advance the operationalization of promising CRT approaches in the form of treatment manuals and associated adherence measures.

Recommendation 14-2: The DoD should convene a conference to achieve consensus among a multiagency (e.g., VA, NIH, and NIDRR), multidisciplinary team of clinicians and researchers to finalize the selection of patient characteristic and outcome variables to be included in experimental and observational CRT research, and to plan a strategy to advance the common definition and operationalization of CRT interventions.

Recommendation 14-3: The DoD should incorporate the selected measures of patient characteristics, outcomes, and defined CRT interventions into ongoing studies (e.g., DVBIC: SCORE!, Millennium, TBI Model System) and develop a comprehensive registry encompassing the existing cohorts and deidentified MHS medical records to allow ongoing evaluation of CRT interventions.

Recommendation 14-4: Using these data sources, the DoD should plan to prospectively evaluate the impact of any policy changes related to CRT delivery and payment within the MHS with respect to outcomes and cost-effectiveness.

Recommendation 14-5: The DoD should collaborate with other research and funding organizations to foster all phases of research and development of CRT treatments for TBI, from pilot phase, to early efficacy research (safety, dose, duration and frequency of exposure, and durability), to large-scale randomized clinical trials, and ultimately, effectiveness and comparative effectiveness studies.

Appendix B

Workshop Agenda

Cognitive Rehabilitation Therapy for Traumatic Brain Injury:
Model Study Protocols and Frameworks to
Advance the State of the Science

October 18–19, 2012
National Academy of Sciences
2101 Constitution Avenue, NW
Washington, DC

DAY 1

9:00–9:15
Welcome and Opening Remarks
Warren Lockette, M.D.
Deputy Assistant Secretary of Defense for Clinical and Program Policy & Chief Medical Officer, TRICARE Management Activity

9:15–9:45
Cognitive Rehabilitation Therapy for Traumatic Brain Injury: Report Overview
Barbara Vickrey, M.D., M.P.H.
Professor and Vice Chair of the Department of Neurology, University of California, Los Angeles

9:45–10:30
Overview of the Translational Pipeline
John Whyte, M.D., Ph.D.
Director, Moss Rehabilitation Research Institute

10:45–11:30
Approaches to Defining and Classifying Rehabilitation Treatments: How Can They Apply to CRT?
Marcel Dijkers, Ph.D.
Senior Investigator, Brain Injury Research Center of Mount Sinai Hospital

11:30–12:00
Setting the Stage for Afternoon Breakout Sessions
John Whyte, M.D., Ph.D.

1:00–2:00
Breakout Session 1: "Modest" Treatment Evidence
Example: Dahlberg, C. A., C. P. Cusick, L. A. Hawley, J. K. Newman, C. E. Morey, C. L. Harrison-Felix, and G. G. Whiteneck. 2007. Treatment efficacy of social communication skills training after traumatic brain injury: A randomized treatment and deferred treatment controlled trial. *Archives of Physical Medicine and Rehabilitation* 88(12):1561–1573.
    Group A: Room NAS 227 (Facilitated by John Whyte)
    Group B: Room NAS 360 (Facilitated by Mary Kennedy)
    Group C: Room NAS Lecture Hall (Facilitated by Hilaire Thompson)

2:00–2:45
Follow-Up Discussion to Breakout Session 1
Moderator: John Whyte, M.D., Ph.D.

3:00–4:00
Breakout Session 2: "Limited" Treatment Evidence
Example: Sohlberg, M. M., K. A. McLaughlin, A. Pavese, A. Heidrich, and M. I. Posner. 2000. Evaluation of attention process training and brain injury education in persons with acquired brain injury. *Journal of Clinical and Experimental Neuropsychology* 22(5):656–676.
    Group A: Room NAS 227 (Facilitated by John Whyte)
    Group B: Room NAS 360 (Facilitated by Mary Kennedy)
    Group C: Room NAS Lecture Hall (Facilitated by Hilaire Thompson)

4:00–4:45
Follow-Up Discussion to Breakout Session 2
Moderator: Mary Kennedy, Ph.D.

4:45–5:00
Closing Remarks
John Whyte, M.D., Ph.D.

DAY 2

9:00–9:30
Recap of Day 1
John Whyte, M.D., Ph.D.

9:30–10:30
Breakout Session 3: "No" Treatment Evidence
Example: Levine, B., I. H. Robertson, L. Clare, G. Carter, J. Hong, B. A. Wilson, J. Duncan, and D. T. Stuss. 2000. Rehabilitation of executive functioning: An experimental-clinical validation of Goal Management Training. *Journal of the International Neuropsychological Society* 6(3):299–312.
    Group A: Room NAS 227 (Facilitated by John Whyte)
    Group B: Room NAS 360 (Facilitated by Mary Kennedy)
    Group C: Room NAS Lecture Hall (Facilitated by Hilaire Thompson)

10:45–11:30
Follow-Up Discussion to Breakout Session 3
Moderator: Hilaire Thompson, Ph.D.

11:30–12:00
Workshop Comments and Synthesis: The Way Forward
John Whyte, M.D., Ph.D.

Appendix C

Biosketches of the Workshop Speakers and Moderators

Marcel Dijkers, Ph.D., studied sociology at the Catholic University of Nijmegen, the Netherlands, and at Wayne State University (WSU) in Detroit, obtaining a Ph.D. in 1978, and he has held a number of research and teaching positions in the Netherlands and the United States. He joined the faculty of the Mount Sinai School of Medicine Department of Rehabilitation Medicine in 1999, and now has the rank of Research Professor. Dr. Dijkers' rehabilitation research interests have been very broad, as evidenced by his more than 100 published papers and chapters, and more than 200 conference presentations. Two areas of focus in terms of diagnosis have been traumatic brain injury (TBI) and spinal cord injury (SCI). He has researched the social and functional consequences of TBI and SCI, the delivery of health services for individuals with these conditions, as well as the determinants of community integration, quality of life, and other outcomes. Research methodology interests have been the measurement of functioning and quality of life, treatment integrity in rehabilitation research, the classification and quantification of treatment, and systematic review/meta-analysis for evidence-based practice. Dr. Dijkers' research has been supported by grants from the National Institute on Disability and Rehabilitation Research and the Centers for Disease Control and Prevention, among others. He is a past president of the *American Congress of Rehabilitation Medicine*, the leading U.S. rehabilitation research organization. He sits on the editorial board of the *Journal of Head Trauma Rehabilitation* and is a regular peer reviewer for a number of other journals. He also serves as grant proposal reviewer for grant-making public and private organizations in the United States and overseas.

Mary R. T. Kennedy, Ph.D., is an Associate Professor in the Speech-Language-Hearing Science Department at the University of Minnesota, Twin Cities. She has more than 30 years of clinical and research experience working with individuals with cognitive and communication disorders as a result of traumatic brain injury (TBI). Dr. Kennedy has published and presented widely on these topics in both peer-reviewed scientific journals and publications aimed at translating evidence into practice. Her research has been funded by grants on the executive functions, language, and metacognition of survivors of TBI and the academic impact of these impairments. Current projects involve translating research evidence into practical assessment and instruction techniques that support individuals with TBI as they transition back to college. Dr. Kennedy chairs the Academy of Neurological Communication Disorders & Sciences (ANCDS) committee that systematically reviews research evidence and develops practice guidelines on managing cognitive and communication disorders after TBI.

Warren Lockette, M.D., is the Deputy Assistant Secretary of Defense for Clinical and Program Policy and the Chief Medical Officer of the TRICARE Management Activity. He is responsible for Department of Defense programs in clinical informatics, military public health, women's health issues, quality management, health promotion and disease prevention, biomedical ethics, mental health policy, patient advocacy, graduate medical education, and patient safety. Dr. Lockette and all of his Military Health System colleagues are dedicated to ensuring that each beneficiary in the Military Health System receives the best health care possible. Dr. Lockette received both his undergraduate and doctor of medicine degrees from the University of Michigan, Ann Arbor. Following postgraduate training at the University of California, he was recruited to the faculty of the Wayne State University School of Medicine, Detroit, and he was a tenured professor of endocrinology and medicine. Dr. Lockette was also appointed Adjunct Associate Professor of Physiology at the University of Michigan and Professor of Medicine and Faculty Fellow of the International House at the University of California, San Diego. In addition to his clinical service, he studies the molecular genetics of complex quantitative traits and human performance in extreme environments. Dr. Lockette has broad experience in operational medicine; he served as a senior advisor to the Commander of the Naval Special Warfare Command and the U.S. Special Operations Command. At Naval Medical Center, San Diego, Dr. Lockette helped guide the growth of the largest military clinical research program in graduate medical education. Most recently, he served as Special Assistant to the Commander, U.S. Navy Fourth Fleet, where he forged partnerships between military and civilian organizations of health care and public health practitioners to provide collaborative humanitarian assistance and disaster relief training in Latin America.

Hilaire Thompson, Ph.D., R.N., FAAN, is an Assistant Professor in the School of Nursing at the University of Washington and a core faculty of the Harborview Injury Prevention and Research Center. Dr. Thompson's research has focused on improving outcomes from traumatic brain injury (TBI). In particular, her efforts have focused on understanding and improving the delivery of health care services to persons with TBI and the use of translational approaches to manage and reduce symptoms following injury. She currently serves as the Clinical Practice Guideline Series editor for the American Association of Neuroscience Nurses. Dr. Thompson earned her Ph.D. in Nursing from the University of Pennsylvania in 2003, after completing her M.S. and Post-M.S. Certificate in Adult Medical-Surgical Nursing and as an Adult Acute Care Nurse Practitioner, respectively from Virginia Commonwealth University. She also received her B.S.N. from Catholic University of America in 1992 and an M.S. in Clinical Epidemiology from the University of Washington in 2008.

Barbara G. Vickrey, M.D., M.P.H., is Professor and Vice Chair of the Department of Neurology at the University of California, Los Angeles (UCLA), where she directs the Health Services Research Program in Neurology. She is also associate director for research at the Greater Los Angeles VA Parkinson Disease Center and an affiliated investigator at the RAND Corporation. Dr. Vickrey's research focuses on translating evidence from clinical trials into routine medical practice and improved patient health outcomes. She led a multisite randomized trial that demonstrated substantially improved quality and better patient and caregiver outcomes from a coordinated care approach to dementia care delivery. Her research has led to enhanced clinical trials for epilepsy and multiple sclerosis by developing widely used instruments to quantify how these patients view their health-related quality of life. Currently, Dr. Vickrey leads an American Heart Association Outcomes Research Center investigating methods to address racial and ethnic disparities in stroke and training postdoctoral fellows in this field of investigation. She received her M.D. from Duke University School of Medicine, and her M.P.H. from UCLA School of Public Health. In 1998, she received the Alice S. Hersh Young Investigator Award from AcademyHealth.

John Whyte, M.D., Ph.D., is a physiatrist and experimental psychologist specializing in traumatic brain injury rehabilitation. He was the founding director of the Moss Rehabilitation Research Institute, begun in 1992, and continues in this position. His research focuses on cognitive impairment and cognitive rehabilitation after brain injury as well as the special methodologic challenges posed by rehabilitation research. Dr. Whyte has received research funding from the National Institutes of Health, the National Institute on Disability and Rehabilitation Research, the Department of the Army, and a number of private foundations. He is the past president of the Association of Academic Physiatrists, former chair of the National Center for Medical Rehabilitation Research's Advisory Board, and past Principal Investigator and Program Director (now Associate Program Director) of the Rehabilitation Medicine Scientist Training Program, a National Institutes of Health–funded program to train psychiatric researchers.